YOUR KNOWLEDGE HAS VALUE

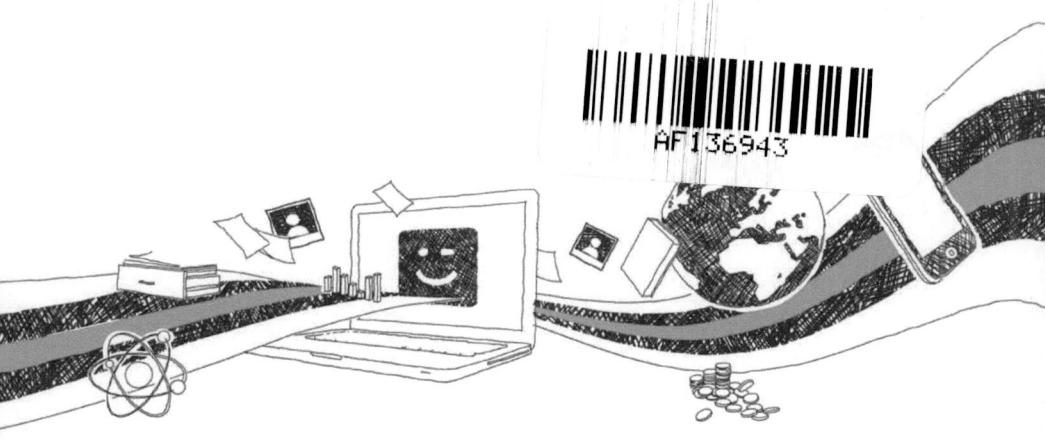

- We will publish your bachelor's and master's thesis, essays and papers

- Your own eBook and book - sold worldwide in all relevant shops

- Earn money with each sale

Upload your text at www.GRIN.com and publish for free

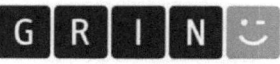

Bibliographic information published by the German National Library:

The German National Library lists this publication in the National Bibliography; detailed bibliographic data are available on the Internet at http://dnb.dnb.de .

Imprint:

Copyright © 2005 GRIN Verlag
Print and binding: Books on Demand GmbH, Norderstedt Germany
ISBN: 9783346161215

This book at GRIN:

https://www.grin.com/document/585136

Dina Were, Jane Amunga

Mental health disorders. Barriers to mental health services among low-income communities in western Kenya

GRIN Verlag

GRIN - Your knowledge has value

Since its foundation in 1998, GRIN has specialized in publishing academic texts by students, college teachers and other academics as e-book and printed book. The website www.grin.com is an ideal platform for presenting term papers, final papers, scientific essays, dissertations and specialist books.

Visit us on the internet:

http://www.grin.com/

http://www.facebook.com/grincom

http://www.twitter.com/grin_com

Kaimosi University College
School of Education and Social Sciences
Department of Foundational Education, Vihiga, Kenya

Barriers To Accessing Mental Health Services Among Low Income Communities In Western Kenya- Qualitative Survey

Dr. Dinah S. Were

Dr. Jane Amunga

Table of Contents

Abstract

Globally mental health illnesses affect more than 25% of all people during their lifetime. Issues on mental health are increasing worldwide and the causes are varied and many. Many young people today are vulnerable as they meet challenges which they are unable to cope with and in many cases leading to mental breakdown. Mental disorders entail a wide range of conditions that may affect mood, thinking, and behavior. Today there are many situations that trigger feelings of worry, anxiety or fear interfering with ones personality. The percentage of people experiencing mental disorders is devastating ranging between 5% - 25% of the population totaling to about 44 million and more in the world. Western Kenya is not exempted and people with mental disorders can be seen in market places, funeral places, on the roads and towns. A qualitative survey was carried out among 114 individuals in western region among them lecturers, medics, university students, social workers and parents to find out barriers to accessing health services in western Kenya. Causes of mental disorders from the research findings were majorly attributed to witchcraft, punishment for evil deeds from God, curses and strange immoral deeds. Among low income communities intervention for those suffering from mental disorders was either postponed or ignored due to the perceptions about the condition. Some resorted to cheaper and crude ways of dealing with the condition which in many cases did not assist clients adequately. Some are too embarrassed to expose their relatives with mental disorders because of the stigma associated with the condition. Other factors contributing to delayed intervention are lack of awareness on where to access help, financial constraints, inadequate trained personnel, lack of drugs in health facilities, scarcity of centers dealing with mental disorders in the country among others. The recommendations were to create awareness on causes of the condition, increase service centers and subsidize the cost of medicines.

Key words: Mental disorders, Well being, low income communities, health services

1 Introduction

Increasing, health and socio-economic burden of mental illnesses and disorders have become a major concern in both developed and developing countries. Globally, it is estimated that more than 450 million people suffer from mental illness or behavioural disorders and one in four families has at least one member with a mental disorder (WHO, 2003). According to WHO (2012), mentally ill people often lack access to education, healthcare and opportunities to earn a decent living, which limits their chances of economic development and deprives them of social protection and recognition within the community. They often have their human rights violated, including being subjected to unhygienic and inhuman living conditions, physical and sexual abuse, neglect, social isolation, as well as stigma and discrimination in health care facilities, in homes and the community at large (Bhugra,1989). The conditions under discussion in this paper include mental illness, depression and extreme aggressive behavior disorders.

The Goal of study
The goal of the study was to find out the barriers to accessing mental health services among low income communities in western Kenya. The survey was carried out through interviews, from a sample of 114 respondents who included lecturers, university students, local leaders, community members, medical personnel and community health workers and spiritual leaders in the western part of Kenya.

Objectives
The objectives were:
i) Causes of mental health disorders in western Kenya

ii) Intervention strategies to mental health disorders in low income communities in western Kenya

iii) Barriers to accessing mental health services among low income communities in western Kenya

2   Causes of mental health disorders

Traditionally families have been seen as contributing to mental illness - either as causing it or aggravating it (Riebschleger, 2001; Marshall, Solomon et al. 2003; Rethink, 2003). They have, at various times in the history of mental illness supported institutionalization (by sending their relatives to psychiatric institutions (Jones, 2002), or been major players in deinstitutionalization (more recently). Many families have assumed a caring role for people with experience of mental illness (Mason, 1996).

In Kenya a pioneer hospital based study was carried out by Omar (2003) in western Kenya. The author found that negative opinions about mental illness were widely held among relatives of mentally ill patients. The respondents had varied opinions on the causation of mental illness. Drug abuse, demons, stress and inheritance were thought to cause mental illness by 38%, 32%, 18% and 10% respectively prayers were suggested as a form of treatment by 76% of the respondents. In western Kenya some of the causes of mental illnesses cited were as follows:

Table 1: Responses on causes of mental disorders

No.	Responses	%
1	Witchcraft or involvement with witches	70
2	Punishment from God for some evil acts	68
3	Curses from people for evil deeds	65
4	Substance abuse	65
5	Demonic forces	60
6	Inherited and runs in the family	45
7	Medical conditions e.g. malaria, tumors	45
8	Abnormal hormonal function in an individual	10

Majority of the respondents prioritized witchcraft as the main cause of mental illness, followed by punishment from God, curses, demonic manifestation and substance abuse as major causes to mental illness. These were followed by inheritance, diseases and abnormal hormonal functions in individuals. The perceptions held traditionally that any form of mental illness is caused by witchcraft, curses and demonic forces causes a lot of stigma towards individuals affected and families. Families blame themselves for the condition and also the communities they live in blame them. The perception about the cause of mental illness to a certain extent determines the treatment strategy.

Many youth in western Kenya cited social causes such as drastic life changes, experiences, family issues, loss of parents/relatives, divorce, drugs and alcohol abuse, loneliness, personality disorders, job loss, failed societal expectations, rejection, false esteem, breakups, and failure to get white collar jobs. Many youth felt depressed from the social issues cited above and expressed concern about inability to access health service due to financial constraints. Joblessness is cited to be one of the leading causes to mental disorders due to financial challenges especially among youths from low income communities.

The youth from able families cited family issues, divorce and societal expectations as major causes of mental illness. Many alluded to the above issues as some of the causes to drug and alcohol abuse which may eventually lead to mental illness and personality disorders.

Some youth also cited low self esteem, breakups in relationships and extreme life changes as some of the causes to depression and mental illnesses.

Some of the medical causes to mental health were prolonged illnesses like cancer, ulcers, migraine headaches, high blood pressure, HIV & AIDS, physical trauma and accidents.

The economic causes to mental illness cited were financial losses and inadequate finances to meet basic needs, medical bills and fees and failure in business.

3   Barriers to mental health services

Both Bower (1998) and Phelan, Bromet et al (1998) report from their respective studies, that family members often try to conceal their relative's mental illness or hospitalization. This is more likely to happen if the person is not living with them, or when the disclosure is avoidable (Phelan, Bromet et al. 1998). The implications of this are that family members in this situation may be more likely to withdraw social contact and are less likely to support their relative with their experience of mental illness (Phelan, Bromet et al. 1998).

The fear may also be due to challenges involved in treating it and that fact that it has no definite treatment. Surprisingly some mentally ill individuals at market places or in communities have always been there since time immemorial. This further makes people believe the condition cannot be cured. There is an unfortunate statement that states "Once mentally ill, always mentally ill". This conclusion is made from the many cases which after treatment, reoccur from time to time. In another study, Ostman and Kjellin

(2002) found that 18 percent of respondents thought that, at times, their relative would be better off dead.

In the Western part of Kenya responses on barriers to accessing mental health services among low income communities were given as follows in the order of priority.

Table 2: Responses on barriers to accessing mental health services

No	Responses	%
1	Inadequate funds, poverty	75
2	Stigma attached to mental health conditions (fear of rejection, negative attitudes towards mental illness)	70
3	No faith in mental health services	68
4	Medication for mental illness is expensive	65
5	Inadequate mental health facilities in the region	65
6	Inadequate trained personnel psychologist, psychiatrists	56
7	Inadequate drugs in health facilities	50
8	Lack of awareness on where to access help	49

Inadequate funds, poverty, stigma attached to mental health conditions, lack of faith in mental health services, high cost of medication and inadequate mental health facilities in western region were major barriers to accessing mental health services. These were followed by inadequate trained personnel, drugs and lack of awareness in the region. The poverty level in most communities in western region is high with most families hardly able to raise one decent meal a day.

On the issue of medical treatment many families cannot afford the medical bills of their family members and in most cases they have to fundraise to pay them. Many (65%) of the respondents raised concern on the high cost of medication for mental illness which makes them opt for cheaper means of treatment. Another shocking revelation by 68% of the respondents was that they did not have faith in medical services for mental illness. They observed that the condition keeps recurring in most of the patients and therefore not effective.

Other responses on barriers to accessing mental health services were 49% of the respondents who cited lack of awareness on mental health facilities. Information on such services has not reached majority of low income communities. In western region there is only one medical facility with admits and treats persons with mental illness.

About 56% of the respondents indicated that there were inadequate trained personnel in the region. The country in general has few psychiatrists and psychologists to handle the rising numbers of people with mental illness. The fear of rejection, negative attitudes, lack of commitment by family members and responsibility over relatives with mental conditions also affects and delays in intervention. The New Zealand discrimination survey (Peterson, Pere et al. 2004) found that 59 percent of people with experience of mental illness reported discrimination from friends and family. This happens a lot among families especially in issues to do with inheritance of property. Many cannot be trusted with family property and are usually left out or given to the guardian. Findings from the New Zealand discrimination survey (Peterson, Pere et al. 2004) suggest that discrimination against people with experience of mental illness is an issue no matter what ethnic or cultural group the person identifies with.

Families share much of the discrimination that people with experience of mental illness face, by being associated with them (Angermeyer, Schulze et al. 2003) and this is discrimination by association (BC Minister of Health's Advisory Council on Mental Health 2002; Ostman and Kjellin, 2002). Many families tend to treat mental illness as a source of shame and embarrassment (Wahl, 1999). Some also indicated that there are no support systems for Persons with mental disorders and inadequate budgetary allocation towards treatment of mental disorders.

Majority of the respondents indicated they lacked funds to take their patients to clinics.

4   Mental illness and perception

Many mental health professionals view families as an 'irritation' (Angermeyer, Schulze et al. 2003). Families are considered by mental health professionals to be interfering and over-protective (Rethink, 2003), and are regarded as being uninformed about mental illness and treatment (Riebschleger, 2001). Family members also report a strained relationship with mental health professionals, who are perceived as being discriminatory towards family members (Angermeyer, Schulze et al. 2003). This may be because the family is perceived by health professionals to be contributing to their relative's mental illness.

It is also perceived to cause poor relations at workplace as colleagues may avoid the individual with mental illness for fear of physical harm. Some respondents also raised concern that individuals with a history of mental illness may not easily get employment and even if employed by chance once discovered the employers find a way of laying them off. There is a wrong perception that such individuals are sick. They are believed to be disabled and unreasonable. This condition is sometimes mistaken for mental retardation which cannot be treated.

One respondent also indicated that they are always careful in the presence of a person with a history of mental illness. One student with a history of mental illness stated that:

> *"most times l feel colleagues never believe me even when l am genuinely happy or sad. They are always suspicious of my behavior. He also added that l find it difficult getting a girlfriend as fellow colleagues warn them of my past and makes them turn me down. They also avoid sharing a room with me for imagining l will harm them".*

He added that even family members were apprehensive of him and treated him with a lot of caution for fear of the unknown. He felt that people around him were observing him all the time for signs of the condition. In Peterson, Pere et al (2004), people with experience of mental illness reported being rejected by friends and family, being called names, being treated as if they were incapable or incompetent, and having family members trying to take control of their lives. He added that his greatest anxiety is the feeling that he might exhibit symptoms of his condition without his conscience. He sometimes appreciates to some extent the concern of people who look out for him. But many times it frustrates him.

He also added that most of the time he found himself explaining his previous history each time he met new friends. But he also observed that whenever he did this some of the friends changed their behavior towards him. He was in a dilemma and found himself lonely and contemplating suicide. Such perception is a result of belief in the stereotypes of people with experience of mental illness leading to prejudice, which in turn leads to discrimination (Schumacher, Corrigan et al. 2003).

Discrimination against, and the stigma of, people with experience of mental illness is widespread (Sayce, 1998; Crisp, Gelder, et al. 2000). It has an impact on the self-esteem (Link, Struening, et al. 2001) and recovery (Perlick, 2001) of people with experience of mental illness, as well as affecting all aspects of people's lives (Penn and Wykes, 2003). Discrimination occurs when a person is treated differently from another person in the same or similar circumstances. For discrimination to occur however, the person with the prejudice must be in a position of power, which must then be exercised (Link and Phelan, 2001). It is clear from the literature that any understanding of stigma and discrimination must include an analysis of power.

Whilst many people in this world face discrimination (on the basis of gender, race, disability amongst others), Gordon, Tantillo et al. (2004) report that discrimination against people with mental illness or intellectual disability seems to evoke the most negative attitudes out of all the disabilities surveyed.

When talking about discrimination and mental illness, Angermeyer, Schulze et al. (2003) report that families tend to talk about their relatives' experiences of discrimination, rather than their own. Some of the literature has recognized that not only are families discriminated against due to their relative's experience of mental illness, they are also an important source of that discrimination (Wahl, 1999a; De Ponte, Bird et al. 2000; Dickerson, Sommerville et al. 2002; Peterson, Pere et al. 2004). Tsang, Tam et al. (2003) concluded in their study based in Hong Kong, that "Stigmatization of patients' families and 'blaming the victim' were so prevalent that even the relatives themselves held those beliefs" (Tsang, Tam et al. 2003 p127). The figures range from 51 percent of people with experience of mental illness reporting discrimination from family (De Ponte, Bird et al. 2000), to 21 percent (Dickerson, Sommerville et al. 2002).

Wahl (1999a) found that discrimination from family was the second most cited form of discrimination. Good, Berenbaum et al. (2000) report that not all families are discriminatory but that those with high levels of 'expressed emotion' are more likely to have negative interactions with their family members. It seems clear, however, that a significant amount of discrimination against those with experience of mental illness comes from family members.

Magliano, Guarneri et al. (2001) surveyed relatives of people with experience of mental illness in Italy and discovered that 68 percent believed that a person with experience of mental illness should be able to vote, 29 percent thought they should be able to have children, and 45 percent that they should be able to work as a babysitter. Forty percent thought that their relative would not recover further.

In Kenya a pioneer hospital based study was carried out by Omar (2003) in western Kenya. The author found that negative opinions about mental illness were widely held among relatives of mentally ill patients. He also found that stigma of mental illness was present in his study population and postulated that it could be higher in the general population. Out of the total study population, (n = 300), the negative opinions held were that the mentally ill are dangerous (53.7%), unpredictable (66.7%), social disgrace (41.7%), hard to talk to (41%), feel different from us (50.3%), had themselves to blame (32%).

Mental illness is one of the most feared conditions among many communities in western Kenya. The fear and beliefs surrounding mental illness are diverse and in some cases due to lack of knowledge about the condition. In many cases individuals prefer other medical conditions to mental illness because of inability to understand and control self. It is compared to death and therefore scary as one of the respondents indicated.

The perceptions affect the individual's social life including marriage as families prohibit their children from marrying from or into families with such history. Such perceptions also affect the assistance offered to individuals suffering from mental illness.

5 Intervention strategies to mental health in low income communities

There is a large number of stereotypes about families of people with experience of mental illness including their being dysfunctional, incompetent, burdened or brave (Banks, 2003). The British Columbia Minister of Health's Advisory Council on Mental Health (2002) reports that these stereotypes have an impact on families of people with experience of mental illness have strained relationships with others, and experience fear, violence, anxiety, conflict, lowered self-esteem and guilt.

While mental health services have changed in the last ten years or so, the 'burden' placed on family members has not lessened (Ostman, Hansson et al. 2000). Angermeyer, Shulze et al. (2003) state succinctly that family members of people with experience of mental illness are characterized by 'responsibility'. That is "they act as the major caretaker, and have a special emotional closeness" (Angermeyer, Shulze, et al. 2003, p602).

The caring role family members sometimes find themselves in has certain implications. In a study by Dore and Romans, (2001) limited to those with bipolar disorder, major costs were incurred as a result of the mental illness. Another challenge is time the family members need to take time off work to care for them. People report a reduction in their income and also difficulties in the relationship with other family members with experience of mental illness (Dore and Romans, 2001). Family members often feel ashamed and helpless (Angermeyer, Schulze et al. 2003), and feel guilty, as if they are the cause of a person's mental illness. They may feel that they somehow have to compensate for their family member's difficulties and social deficits (Perlick, Rosenheck et al. 2001).

This also applies here in western Kenya among communities with mental illness. They blame themselves for the mental illness of their member of family. This is so especially where it is believed the family was involved in some evil deeds, or cursed or punished

11

by God for some evil acts. The family is also stigmatized and in some cases segregated. The advice from elders, witchdoctors and medicine men revolves around various rituals in the effort of cleansing family members and home in general of those deeds to appease the gods or ancestors. Responses on intervention strategies for relatives with the condition are as indicated in the table below.

Table 3: Responses on intervention strategies

SNo.	Responses on intervention strategies among low income communities	%
1	Visits spiritual people	95
2	Visits witch doctors	76
3	Visits mental health services clinics	50
4	Have been involved in rituals by elders	40
5	Have visited psychiatrist and psychologist	10
6	Confinement in homes	10

Source researcher, 2019

In Kenya a pioneer hospital based study was carried out by Omar (2003) in western Kenya on the opinions about treatment of mentally ill. The author found that negative opinions about mental illness were widely held among relatives of mentally ill patients. Knowledge on mental illness treatment was remarkably high with 96% of the respondents believing that medical treatment is necessary, 80% believed that the mentally ill patients will improve if treated and 62.7% believed that mentally ill patients will eventually recover. From this review, it is clear that negative attitudes towards mental illness and the mentally ill exist in the general population. Prayers were suggested as a form of treatment by 76% of the respondents. This stigma affects all aspects of patients' life. It is directed to them not only by lay people but medical professionals as well.

The challenge with this condition is that many times one will not know when it occurs and so they have to depend on their close friends and relatives to make them aware either to take rest, leave or treatment. Depending on the severity of the mental illness one have to depend on relatives all their life for everything. There are a few individuals who are on medication for mental illness who have maintained their jobs with the help

12

of colleagues at workplace. The role of their close colleagues is to monitor their behavior for signs of stress and advice accordingly. This involves a lot of commitment and love for such individuals. The colleagues may be required to cover up for their behavior and take up duties while their colleague is on leave or off duty. It also takes an understanding employer to ensure the welfare of such employees and take appropriate action whenever need arises.

This topic has been researched on more in the west than in Africa yet it has been demonstrated that it not only affects patients' quality of life but their health seeking behaviors as well. Studies on psychiatric morbidity in Kenya have clearly demonstrated the illness burden, Ndetei and Muhangi in (1979). They studied 140 rural walk-in clinic patients and found that 20% suffered psychiatric illnesses; especially depression. Sebit (1996) assessed 186 patients attending primary health care facilities and found an overall prevalence rate of psychiatric disorders at 0.43%. As cited earlier, further stigma research in the general population in Kenya is necessary.

Majority (95%) of respondents from low income communities indicated that when an individual falls mentally ill the first thing was to seek for prayers from spiritual leaders to remove demons purportedly haunting the person. They believe mental illness is usually associated with demonic forces. They also believe majority of mental illnesses can be cured if the right spiritual intervention is applied. They also cited cases where the situation got worse or reoccurred especially if false or wrong spiritual leaders were used.

Witchdoctors were also consulted in case of mental illness as cited by 76% of the respondents. The respondents indicated that witchdoctors were able to establish the evil forces causing the mental illness. Many of the respondents indicated that this is not done openly because it was not viewed positively by the society. It was done secretly and it involved a lot of conditions. Some indicated that they did not have a lot of trust in witchdoctors as the mental illness reoccurred and in some cases worse than before.

Some 50% of the respondents indicated that some mentally ill individuals were taken to medical clinics in the initial stages of the condition. The respondents also added that in most cases individuals had to be on medication for some time which became expensive for low income communities. Although they indicated mental illness due to infections was well handled in general medical clinics. In most cases once an individual accepted the medication they would register and collect their own medication.

A few (10%) of the respondents indicated that some of the mentally ill individuals were taken to psychologists if funds were available. Another 10% indicated mentally ill individuals were confined in homes especially if they were aggressive and causing harm to the public. Some were locked up in chains or rooms and only feed through windows or openings. They did not have showers or clean clothes. This was usually the last option after all the other intervention strategies had failed.

6   Conclusion

Barriers to mental health were diverse and were pegged on the cause of the mental illness or disorder and the perception of the family and community in general. Intervention strategies depended on the financial ability of the family and level of mental illness. Mental health services were few and the cost of medication was high. Majority of people did not believe in the medical treatment of mental illness.

Recommendations

- Increase awareness on mental health conditions
- Increase awareness on the mental health facilities available in the country
- Increase budgetary allocation towards mental health services
- Increase service centers in the country
- Train more personnel in mental health issues
- Subsidize the cost on medication
- Form support systems for mental health
- Increase rehabilitation centers

7 References

Angermeyer, M., B. Schulze, et al. (2003). "Courtesy stigma: A focus group study of relatives of schizophrenia patients." Social Psychiatry and Psychiatric Epidemiology 38: 593-602.

Banks, M. (2003). "Disability in the family life: A life span perspective." Cultural Diversity and Ethnic Minority Psychology 9(4): 367-384.

BC Minister of Health's Advisory Council on Mental Health (2002). Discrimination against people with mental illnesses and their families: Changing attitudes, opening minds: Executive summary and major recommendations. Vancouver, Canadian Mental Health Association.

Bower, B. (1998). "Family shroud for the mentally ill." Science News 153(10): 152.

Corrigan, P., G. Bodenhausen, et al. (2003). "Demonstrating translational research for mental health services: An example of stigma research." Mental Health Services Research 5(2): 79-88.

Corrigan, P., L. River, et al. (2001). "Three strategies for changing attributions about severe mental illness." Schizophrenia Bulletin 27(2): 187-195.

Crisp, A., M. Gelder, et al. (2000). "Stigmatisation of people with mental illness." British Journal of Psychiatry 177: 4-7.

De Ponte, P., L. Bird, et al. (2000). Pull yourself together! A survey of the stigma and discrimination faced by people who experience mental distress. London, The Mental Health Foundation.

Dickerson, F., J. Sommerville, et al. (2002). "Mental illness stigma: An impediment to psychiatric rehabilitation." Psychiatric Rehabilitation Skills 6(2): 186-200.

Dore, G. and S. Romans (2001). "Impact of bipolar affective disorder on family and partners." Journal of Affective Disorders 67(1-3): 147-158.

Durie, M. (1994). "Maori Psychiatric Admissions: Patterns and Policies". Social Dimensions of Health and Disease: New Zealand Perspectives. J. Spicer, A. Trlin and J. Walton. Palmerston North, Dunmore Press: 323-335.

Durie, M. (1997). "Whanau Whanaungatanga". Mai i Rangiatea; Maori Wellbeing and Development. P. Te Whaiti, M. McCarthy and A. Durie. Auckland, Auckland University Press: 1-24.

Dyall, L. (1997). "Maori". Mental Health in New Zealand from a Public Health Perspective. P. Ellis and S. Collings. Wellington, Ministry of Health: 85-103.

Good, T., H. Berenbaum, et al. (2000). "Residential caregiver attitudes toward seriously mentally ill persons." Psychiatry 63(1): 23-33.

Gordon, P., J. Tantillo, et al. (2004). "Attitudes regarding interpersonal relationships with persons with mental illness and mental retardation." Journal of Rehabilitation 70(1): 50-56.

Gordon, S. (2005). The Power of Contact Wellington, Case Consulting

Jones, D. (2002). "Madness, the family and psychiatry." Critical Social Policy 22(2): 247-272.

Link, B. and J. Phelan (2001). "Conceptualizing stigma." Annual Review of Sociology 27: 363-385.

Link, B., E. Struening, et al. (2001). "The consequences of stigma for the self-esteem of people with mental illnesses." Psychiatric Services 52(12): 1621-1626.

Magliano, L., A. Fiorillo, et al. (2004). "Beliefs about schizophrenia in Italy: A comparative nationwide survey of the general public, mental health professionals, and patients' relatives." Canadian Journal of Psychiatry 49(5): 323-331.

Magliano, L., M. Guarneri, et al. (2001). "A multicenter Italian study of patients' relatives' beliefs about schizophrenia." Psychiatric Services 52(11): 1528-1530.

Marshall, T., P. Solomon, et al. (2003). "Provider and family beliefs regarding the causes of severe mental illness." Psychiatric Quarterly 74(3): 223-236.

Mason, K. (1996). Inquiry under section 47 of the Health and Disability Services Act 1993 in respect of certain mental health services: Report of the ministerial inquiry to the Minister of Health Hon Jenny Shipley. Wellington, Minister of Health.

Mental Health Commission (1998). Blueprint for mental health services in New Zealand: How things need to be. Wellington, Mental Health Commission.

Ministry of Health (1998). Whaia Te Whanaungatanga: Oranga Whanau The Wellbeing of Whanau. Wellington, Ministry of Health.

Ostman, M., L. Hansson, et al. (2000). "Family burden, participation in care and mental health - an 11 year comparison of the situation of relatives to compulsorily and voluntarily admitted patients." International Journal of Social Psychiatry 46(3): 191-200.

Ostman, M. and L. Kjellin (2002). "Stigma by association: Psychological factors in relatives of people with mental illness." British Journal of Psychiatry 181: 494-498.

Penn, D. and T. Wykes (2003). "Stigma, discrimination and mental illness." Journal of Mental Health 12(3): 203-208.

Perlick, D. (2001). "Special section on stigma as a barrier to recovery." Psychiatric Services 52(12): 1613-1614.

Perlick, D., R. Rosenheck, et al. (2001). "Adverse effects of perceived stigma on social adaptation of persons diagnosed with bipolar affective disorder." Psychiatric Services 52(12): 1627-1632.

Peterson, D., L. Pere, et al. (2004). Respect costs nothing: A survey of discrimination faced by people with experience of mental illness in Aotearoa New Zealand. Wellington, Mental Health Foundation.

Phelan, J., E. Bromet, et al. (1998). "Psychiatric illness and family stigma." Schizophrenia Bulletin 24(1): 115-126.

Phillips, M., V. Pearson, et al. (2002). "Stigma and expressed emotion: a study of people with schizophrenia and their family members in China." British Journal of Psychiatry 181: 488-493.

Reinke, R., P. Corrigan, et al. (2004). "Examining two aspects of contact on the stigma of mental illness." Journal of Social and Clinical Psychology 23(3): 377-389.

Rethink (2003). Who cares? The experiences of mental health carers accessing services and information. London, Rethink.

Riebschleger, J. (2001). "What do mental health professionals really think of family members of mental health patients?" American Journal of Orthopsychiatry 71(4): 466-472.

Sayce, L. (1998). "Stigma, discrimination and social exclusion: What's in a word?" Journal of Mental Health 7(4): 331-343.

Scheurich (2002). "Moral attitudes and mental disorders." The Hasting Center Report 32(2): 14-21.

Schumacher, M., P. Corrigan, et al. (2003). "Examining cues that signal mental illness stigma." Journal of Social and Clinical Psychology 22(5): 467-476.

Tsang, H., P. Tam, et al. (2003). "Sources of burdens on families of individuals with mental illness." International Journal of Rehabilitation Research 26(2): 123-130.

Wahl, O. (1999). "Mental health consumers' experience of stigma." Schizophrenia Bulletin 25(3): 467-478.

Wahl, O. (1999a). Telling is risky business: The experience of mental illness stigma. New Jersey, Rutgers University Press.

YOUR KNOWLEDGE HAS VALUE

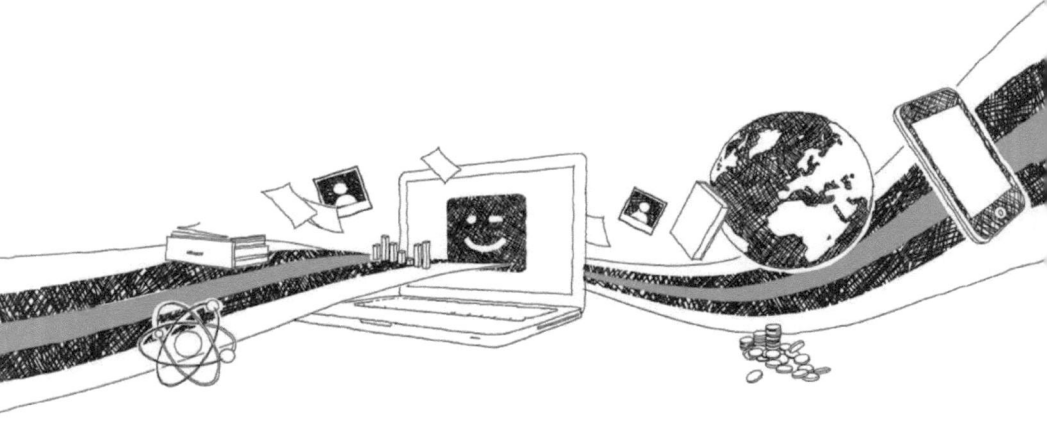

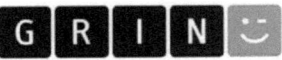